EAT TO BEAT COPD

Healthy Eating Recipes And Menu Plans For The Respiratory System + Particularities For Patients With Chronic Obstructive Pulmonary Disease

DR. LONDYN DELANEY

Table of Contents

Introductory

COPD stands for Chronic Obstructive Pulmonary Disease. It's a chronic inflammatory lung disease that causes obstructed airflow from the lungs. The primary symptoms include difficulty breathing, coughing, wheezing, and tightness in the chest. COPD typically worsens over time and is often caused by long-term exposure to irritating gases or particulate matter, most commonly from cigarette smoke.

Causes and Risk Factors:

COPD is primarily caused by long-term exposure to irritating gases or particulate matter that damage the lungs and airways. The most common risk factor is smoking cigarettes or other forms of tobacco. Other causes and risk factors include:

- **Smoking**: Cigarette smoking is the leading cause of COPD. The majority of people with COPD are current or former smokers.

- **Environmental Exposure**: Long-term exposure to air pollutants such as chemical fumes, dust, or vapors in the workplace can contribute to COPD. This is more common in certain occupations like coal mining, construction work, or those involving chemical production.

- **Genetic Factors**: A small percentage of people with COPD have a genetic predisposition known as alpha-1 antitrypsin deficiency. This genetic disorder can lead to early onset COPD, especially in individuals who smoke or have significant exposure to lung irritants.

- **Indoor Air Pollution**: Exposure to indoor air pollutants such as biomass fuels (used for cooking and heating in poorly ventilated homes) can contribute to COPD, particularly in developing countries.

• **Age**: COPD most commonly develops in people over the age of 40, and the risk increases with age.

• **Respiratory Infections**: Severe respiratory infections during childhood or adulthood can increase the risk of developing COPD.

• **Family History**: A family history of COPD can increase your susceptibility to developing the condition, especially if combined with other risk factors like smoking.

It's important to note that while these factors increase the likelihood of developing COPD, not everyone exposed to them will develop the disease. Quitting smoking and reducing exposure to lung irritants are crucial steps in preventing COPD or slowing its progression. Early detection and management of COPD can significantly improve outcomes and quality of life for individuals affected by the condition.

CHAPTER ONE
Symptoms And Diagnosis

The symptoms of COPD typically develop slowly over time, and they can vary in severity. The main symptoms include:

• **Shortness of Breath**: This is often the earliest symptom, initially occurring during physical exertion and later progressing to occur during rest.

• **Chronic Cough**: A persistent cough that may produce mucus (sputum) that may be clear, white, yellow, or greenish.

• **Wheezing**: A whistling or squeaky sound when you breathe.

• **Chest Tightness**: A feeling of constriction or pressure in the chest.

• **Frequent Respiratory Infections**: COPD can make you more susceptible to respiratory infections such as colds, flu, and pneumonia.

• **Fatigue**: Feeling tired or lacking energy, especially during physical activity.

Diagnosis of COPD usually involves several steps:

• **Medical History**: Your doctor will ask about your symptoms, smoking history, exposure to lung irritants, and any family history of lung disease.

• **Physical Examination**: This includes listening to your lungs with a stethoscope to check for abnormal breath sounds.

• **Lung Function Tests**: The most common test is spirometry, which measures how much air you can inhale and exhale and how quickly you can exhale. This test helps determine the severity of airflow obstruction and is essential for diagnosing COPD.

• **Imaging Tests**: Chest X-rays or CT scans may be used to rule out other lung conditions or to assess the extent of lung damage caused by COPD.

• **Blood Tests**: These may be done to rule out other conditions or to check for oxygen levels in the blood.

Once diagnosed, COPD is categorized into stages based on the severity of airflow limitation according to spirometry results. This helps guide treatment and management strategies. Early diagnosis and appropriate management can help slow the progression of COPD and improve quality of life.

Importance Of Nutrition In Managing COPD

Nutrition plays a crucial role in managing COPD (Chronic Obstructive Pulmonary Disease) because it can directly impact lung function, overall health, and quality of life for individuals with this condition. Here are several key reasons why nutrition is important in managing COPD:

• **Maintaining Healthy Body Weight**: COPD can lead to weight loss and muscle wasting due to increased energy expenditure during breathing and decreased appetite. Proper nutrition helps maintain a healthy weight, which is important for overall strength and respiratory muscle function.

• **Energy Requirements**: People with COPD often have increased energy needs due to the extra effort required for breathing. Adequate calorie intake ensures sufficient energy levels to support daily activities and reduce fatigue.

• **Nutrient Requirements**: COPD can affect the body's ability to absorb nutrients, particularly if lung disease leads to reduced physical activity or if medications affect appetite. Proper nutrition ensures adequate intake of essential nutrients such as vitamins (especially vitamin D and B vitamins), minerals (like calcium and magnesium), and antioxidants (such as vitamin C and E), which are important for immune function and reducing inflammation.

• **Muscle Strength and Respiratory Function**: Protein is crucial for maintaining and repairing muscles, including respiratory muscles. Adequate protein intake supports muscle strength and endurance, which can improve breathing efficiency.

• **Immune Function**: Good nutrition supports a healthy immune system, which is important for preventing and fighting respiratory infections that can exacerbate COPD symptoms.

• **Managing Symptoms and Exacerbations**: Certain dietary choices, such as avoiding excessive salt (sodium) intake, can help manage symptoms like shortness of breath and reduce fluid retention, which can worsen breathing difficulties during exacerbations.

• **Breathing Efficiency**: Some foods, such as those rich in omega-3 fatty acids (found in fish like salmon and sardines), may have anti-inflammatory effects that can help reduce inflammation in the lungs and improve breathing function.

• **Hydration**: Staying well-hydrated helps keep mucus thin and easier to clear from the airways, which can reduce coughing and improve breathing comfort.

• **Medication Effectiveness**: Proper nutrition can enhance the effectiveness of medications used to manage COPD symptoms and reduce the risk of side effects.

Managing nutrition for COPD often involves working with healthcare professionals, such as dietitians or nutritionists, to develop a personalized plan that meets individual needs and preferences. This plan may include strategies to ensure adequate nutrient intake, maintain a healthy weight, and optimize energy levels to support daily activities and respiratory function.

Common Nutritional Deficiencies In COPD Patients

Nutritional deficiencies are common among COPD (Chronic Obstructive Pulmonary Disease) patients due to various factors related to the disease itself and its management. Some of the most prevalent nutritional deficiencies in COPD patients include:

• **Protein**: Many COPD patients experience muscle wasting and weight loss due to increased energy expenditure during breathing and reduced physical activity. Protein deficiency can exacerbate muscle weakness and respiratory muscle fatigue, impairing overall respiratory function.

• **Vitamin D**: Deficiency in vitamin D is common among COPD patients, partly due to limited sun exposure (often exacerbated by reduced outdoor activity) and impaired vitamin D synthesis in the skin. Vitamin D deficiency can impact bone health and immune function, potentially worsening COPD outcomes.

• **Antioxidants (Vitamin C and E)**: COPD is associated with increased oxidative stress and inflammation in the lungs. Antioxidants such as vitamin C and E help neutralize free radicals and reduce inflammation. Deficiencies in these antioxidants may contribute to exacerbations of COPD symptoms.

• **Magnesium**: Magnesium deficiency can occur in COPD patients, possibly due to increased urinary loss or poor intake. Magnesium is important for muscle function and relaxation, including respiratory muscles, and deficiency may contribute to muscle weakness and fatigue.

• **Omega-3 Fatty Acids**: COPD patients may have lower levels of omega-3 fatty acids, which have anti-inflammatory properties. Low omega-3 intake may exacerbate inflammation in the lungs and contribute to worsening respiratory symptoms.

• **Calcium**: Calcium deficiency can occur in COPD patients, especially if they have osteoporosis or are on corticosteroid therapy, which can increase calcium excretion. Calcium is essential for bone health, and deficiency can lead to increased risk of fractures.

• **B Vitamins**: Certain B vitamins, such as vitamin B6 and B12, are important for energy metabolism and nerve function. Deficiencies in these vitamins can contribute to fatigue and worsen overall energy levels in COPD patients.

Managing these nutritional deficiencies is crucial for optimizing COPD management and improving quality of life. It often involves dietary adjustments, possibly with the guidance of a healthcare professional or dietitian, and in some cases, supplementation may be necessary to correct deficiencies effectively.

CHAPTER TWO
Principles Of A COPD Diet Plan

A COPD diet plan aims to support overall health, manage symptoms, and optimize nutrition for individuals with Chronic Obstructive Pulmonary Disease (COPD). Here are some key principles to consider when developing a COPD diet plan:

• **Maintain a Healthy Weight**: Many COPD patients struggle with maintaining their weight due to increased energy expenditure and reduced appetite. It's important to ensure adequate calorie intake to prevent weight loss and muscle wasting, while avoiding excessive weight gain that can strain respiratory function.

• **Focus on Balanced Nutrition**: Emphasize a diet rich in fruits, vegetables, whole grains, lean proteins, and healthy fats. This provides essential nutrients, vitamins, and minerals needed for overall health and immune function.

• **Protein-Rich Foods**: Include adequate protein sources such as lean meats, poultry, fish, eggs, dairy products, legumes, and nuts. Protein is crucial for maintaining muscle strength, including respiratory muscles, and supporting overall physical function.

• **Omega-3 Fatty Acids**: Incorporate foods rich in omega-3 fatty acids, such as fatty fish (salmon, mackerel, sardines), flaxseeds, chia seeds, and walnuts. Omega-3s have anti-inflammatory properties that may help reduce inflammation in the lungs.

• **Hydration**: Drink plenty of fluids, primarily water, throughout the day to keep mucus thin and easier to clear from the airways. Avoid excessive caffeine and alcohol, as they can contribute to dehydration.

• **Small, Frequent Meals**: Eating smaller, more frequent meals throughout the day can help prevent bloating and discomfort, especially for COPD patients who may experience shortness of breath with larger meals.

• **Limit Sodium**: Reduce sodium intake to help prevent fluid retention and bloating, which can worsen breathing difficulties. Avoid processed and salty foods, and instead, season foods with herbs and spices.

• **Vitamin D and Calcium**: Ensure adequate intake of vitamin D-rich foods (fatty fish, fortified dairy products, egg yolks) and calcium-rich foods (dairy products, leafy greens, fortified plant-based milks) to support bone health.

• **Fiber-Rich Foods**: Include plenty of fiber from fruits, vegetables, whole grains, and legumes to support digestive health and maintain regular bowel movements.

• **Consider Individual Needs**: Tailor the diet plan to individual preferences, nutritional needs, and any specific dietary restrictions or allergies.

Work with a registered dietitian or healthcare provider to develop a personalized COPD diet plan that addresses specific nutritional needs, medication interactions, and overall health goals.

By following these principles, individuals with COPD can support their respiratory function, maintain muscle strength, manage symptoms effectively, and improve their overall quality of life. Regular monitoring and adjustments to the diet plan may be necessary based on changes in health status or treatment regimens.

Foods To Include And Avoid

When creating a diet plan for COPD (Chronic Obstructive Pulmonary Disease), it's important to focus on foods that support overall health, provide essential nutrients, and help manage symptoms. Here are some specific foods to include and avoid:

Foods to Include:

• **Lean Proteins**: Such as chicken, turkey, fish (especially fatty fish like salmon and trout for omega-3s), lean cuts of beef or pork, eggs, low-fat dairy products, legumes (beans, lentils), and tofu. Protein is important for maintaining muscle strength, including respiratory muscles.

• **Fruits and Vegetables**: Choose a variety of colorful fruits and vegetables, aiming for at least 5 servings per day. They provide vitamins, minerals, antioxidants, and fiber.

Examples include berries, citrus fruits, apples, leafy greens, tomatoes, bell peppers, broccoli, carrots, and sweet potatoes.

• **Whole Grains**: Opt for whole grains such as oats, quinoa, brown rice, whole wheat bread, and whole grain pasta. They provide fiber, which supports digestive health and helps maintain stable energy levels.

• **Healthy Fats**: Include sources of healthy fats, such as olive oil, avocado, nuts (like almonds, walnuts), seeds (flaxseeds, chia seeds), and fatty fish. Omega-3 fatty acids from fish and seeds have anti-inflammatory properties that may benefit lung health.

• **Fluids**: Stay well-hydrated with water primarily. Herbal teas and diluted fruit juices can also contribute to hydration. Keeping mucus thin and easy to clear helps manage symptoms.

• **Calcium and Vitamin D Sources**: Include dairy products (if tolerated), fortified plant-based milks, fortified cereals, fatty fish, egg yolks, and sunlight exposure (for vitamin D synthesis).

• **Fiber-Rich Foods**: Whole grains, fruits, vegetables, legumes, and nuts/seeds provide fiber that supports digestive health and regular bowel movements.

Foods to Avoid or Limit:

• **Sodium**: Reduce intake of high-sodium foods like processed meats (sausages, bacon), canned soups, salty snacks (chips, pretzels), and fast food. High sodium intake can lead to fluid retention and worsen symptoms.

• **Processed Foods**: Minimize intake of processed and packaged foods that are high in unhealthy fats, sugars, and additives. They often lack nutritional value and can contribute to inflammation.

• **Caffeine and Alcohol**: Limit caffeine and alcohol consumption as they can contribute to dehydration, which can worsen mucus production and respiratory symptoms.

• **Gas-Producing Foods**: Some people with COPD may find that certain foods like beans, cabbage, and carbonated beverages can cause bloating and discomfort. Pay attention to how these foods affect you individually.

• **Heavy Meals**: Large meals can make breathing more difficult. Instead, opt for smaller, more frequent meals throughout the day.

• **Allergens or Sensitivities**: Avoid foods that trigger allergies or sensitivities, as they can worsen respiratory symptoms and inflammation.

• **Eat Mindfully**: Take your time to eat slowly and chew food thoroughly to reduce discomfort and bloating.

• **Monitor Fluid Intake**: Aim for adequate hydration throughout the day, but avoid excessive fluid intake just before bedtime to minimize nighttime trips to the bathroom.

• **Individualize Your Diet**: Work with a healthcare provider or dietitian to personalize your diet plan based on your specific nutritional needs, health status, and any dietary restrictions.

By focusing on nutrient-dense foods, managing portion sizes, and being mindful of dietary triggers, individuals with COPD can better manage their symptoms, support overall health, and improve quality of life.

Recommended Daily Intake Of Nutrients

The recommended daily intake of nutrients for individuals with COPD (Chronic Obstructive Pulmonary Disease) is generally similar to that recommended for the general population, with some considerations for managing symptoms and supporting overall health. Here's a general guideline for daily nutrient intake:

<u>*Macronutrients:*</u>

Protein:

• Aim for 1.2 to 1.7 grams of protein per kilogram of body weight per day. This helps support muscle strength and repair, including respiratory muscles.

• Example: For a person weighing 70 kg (154 lbs), this would be approximately 84 to 119 grams of protein per day.

Carbohydrates:

• Carbohydrates should make up about 45-65% of total daily calories. Focus on complex carbohydrates from whole grains, fruits, and vegetables for sustained energy.

Fats:

• Limit saturated fats and trans fats. Instead, include sources of healthy fats like omega-3 fatty acids (from fatty fish, flaxseeds, chia seeds) and monounsaturated fats (from olive oil, avocados, nuts).

Micronutrients:

Vitamins:

• **Vitamin D**: Aim for 600-800 IU (International Units) per day. This can be obtained from sunlight (limited exposure), fatty fish (salmon, mackerel), fortified dairy products, and supplements if necessary.

• **Vitamin C**: Aim for 75-90 mg per day for women and men, respectively. Good sources include citrus fruits, berries, tomatoes, and leafy greens.

• **Vitamin E**: Aim for 15 mg per day. Sources include nuts, seeds, and vegetable oils.

• **B Vitamins**: Include sources of vitamin B6 (1.3-1.7 mg/day), vitamin B12 (2.4 mcg/day), and folate (400 mcg/day). These are important for energy metabolism and nerve function.

Minerals:

• **Calcium**: Aim for 1000-1200 mg per day for adults, depending on age and gender. Sources include dairy products (if tolerated), fortified plant-based milks, leafy greens, and supplements if necessary.

• **Magnesium**: Aim for 320-420 mg per day for women and men, respectively. Good sources include nuts, seeds, whole grains, and green leafy vegetables.

• **Potassium**: Aim for 3500-4700 mg per day. Sources include bananas, oranges, potatoes, and leafy greens.

Fluids:

• Stay well-hydrated with water primarily. Aim for 8-10 cups (about 2-2.5 liters) of fluids per day, adjusting for individual needs and climate.

Additional Considerations:

• **Fiber**: Aim for 25-30 grams of fiber per day from fruits, vegetables, whole grains, and legumes to support digestive health.

• **Sodium**: Limit sodium intake to less than 2300 mg per day (or even lower if recommended by healthcare provider) to help manage fluid balance and reduce bloating.

• **Omega-3 Fatty Acids**: Aim for at least 250-500 mg of EPA and DHA combined per day, primarily from fatty fish or supplements if needed.

Individual nutrient needs may vary based on factors such as age, sex, weight, activity level, and specific health conditions. It's important to consult with a registered dietitian or healthcare provider to tailor nutrient intake recommendations to your individual needs and to ensure optimal management of COPD symptoms and overall health.

CHAPTER THREE
Sample Meal Plans For Different Stages Of COPD

Creating sample meal plans for different stages of COPD (Chronic Obstructive Pulmonary Disease) involves tailoring nutritional intake to support energy needs, manage symptoms, and maintain overall health. Here are sample meal plans for three stages of COPD severity: mild, moderate, and severe.

Mild COPD (Stage 1):

Breakfast:

- Oatmeal topped with berries and a sprinkle of ground flaxseeds
- Scrambled eggs with spinach
- Whole grain toast with avocado

Morning Snack:

• Greek yogurt with sliced almonds and a drizzle of honey

Lunch:

- Grilled chicken salad with mixed greens, cherry tomatoes, cucumber, and olive oil vinaigrette
- Whole grain roll

Afternoon Snack:

• Apple slices with almond butter

Dinner:

- Baked salmon with quinoa and steamed broccoli
- Mixed green salad with a variety of vegetables

Evening Snack:

• Air-popped popcorn seasoned with herbs

Moderate COPD (Stage 2):

Breakfast:

- Smoothie with spinach, berries, banana, Greek yogurt, and chia seeds
- Whole grain toast with avocado or nut butter

Morning Snack:

• Cottage cheese with pineapple chunks

Lunch:

- Turkey and avocado wrap with whole grain tortilla, lettuce, and tomato
- Carrot sticks with hummus

Afternoon Snack:

• Mixed nuts (almonds, walnuts, pistachios)

Dinner:

- Grilled shrimp skewers with quinoa pilaf (mixed with vegetables)
- Steamed asparagus

Evening Snack:

• Whole grain crackers with cheese

Severe COPD (Stage 3-4):

Breakfast:

- Scrambled eggs with cheese and spinach
- Whole grain toast with nut butter

Morning Snack:

• Smoothie with protein powder, banana, almond milk, and spinach

Lunch:

- Minestrone soup with added beans and vegetables
- Whole grain roll

Afternoon Snack:

• Avocado with whole grain crackers

Dinner:

- Baked chicken breast with sweet potato mash and steamed green beans
- Spinach salad with strawberries and balsamic vinaigrette

Evening Snack:

• Greek yogurt with honey and granola

General Tips for Meal Planning in COPD:

• **Balanced Nutrition**: Ensure each meal includes a balance of carbohydrates, protein, and healthy fats to support energy levels and muscle strength.

• **Small, Frequent Meals**: Eating smaller meals throughout the day can reduce bloating and discomfort associated with fullness, making breathing easier.

• **Hydration**: Stay well-hydrated with water and other fluids throughout the day to keep mucus thin and easy to clear.

• **Fiber**: Include fiber-rich foods like fruits, vegetables, and whole grains to support digestive health.

• **Individual Needs**: Adjust portion sizes and specific food choices based on individual preferences, dietary restrictions, and nutritional needs.

Consulting with a registered dietitian or healthcare provider can help customize meal plans based on specific nutritional requirements, COPD severity, and any other health considerations.

Regular monitoring and adjustment of dietary plans may be necessary to optimize nutritional intake and manage COPD symptoms effectively.

Snack Ideas And Quick Meals Recipes

Here are some snack ideas and quick meal recipes that are convenient and nutritious, suitable for individuals managing COPD (Chronic Obstructive Pulmonary Disease):

Snack Ideas:

Greek Yogurt Parfait:

• Layer Greek yogurt with berries (like strawberries or blueberries) and a sprinkle of granola or nuts.

Smoothie:

• Blend spinach, banana, almond milk (or yogurt), and a scoop of protein powder for added nutrition.

Apple Slices with Nut Butter:

• Slice apples and dip them in almond butter or peanut butter for a satisfying snack.

Hummus and Veggie Sticks:

• Dip carrot sticks, cucumber slices, and bell pepper strips in hummus for a crunchy and nutritious snack.

Whole Grain Crackers with Cheese:

• Pair whole grain crackers with slices of cheese (like cheddar or Swiss) for a quick and protein-packed snack.

Trail Mix:

• Combine nuts (like almonds, walnuts) with dried fruits (such as apricots or raisins) for a portable snack.

Rice Cakes with Avocado:

• Spread mashed avocado on rice cakes and sprinkle with a pinch of sea salt and pepper.

Cottage Cheese with Pineapple:

• Enjoy cottage cheese with pineapple chunks for a balanced snack.

Quick Meal Recipes:

Vegetable Stir-Fry:

• Heat olive oil in a pan and stir-fry mixed vegetables (bell peppers, broccoli, carrots) with tofu or chicken strips.

• Season with soy sauce, garlic, and ginger. Serve over brown rice or quinoa.

Tuna Salad Wrap:

• Mix canned tuna with Greek yogurt, diced celery, and a squeeze of lemon juice.

• Spread on a whole grain tortilla, add lettuce leaves, roll up, and enjoy.

Caprese Salad:

• Layer sliced tomatoes, fresh mozzarella cheese, and basil leaves on a plate.

• Drizzle with balsamic glaze and olive oil. Season with salt and pepper to taste.

Egg and Vegetable Scramble:

• Whisk eggs with a splash of milk. Sauté diced vegetables (spinach, tomatoes, mushrooms) in olive oil until tender.

• Pour in the eggs and scramble until cooked through. Serve with whole grain toast.

Chicken and Vegetable Soup:

• In a pot, combine diced chicken breast, mixed vegetables (like carrots, celery, and peas), low-sodium chicken broth, and herbs (such as thyme and parsley).

• Simmer until vegetables are tender and chicken is cooked. Season to taste.

Quinoa Salad:

• Cook quinoa according to package instructions. Let it cool.

• Mix with diced cucumber, cherry tomatoes, black beans, and a dressing made from olive oil, lemon juice, and herbs (like cilantro or parsley).

Avocado Toast:

• Mash ripe avocado with a fork and spread on whole grain toast.

• Top with sliced tomatoes, a sprinkle of sea salt, and a drizzle of olive oil.

• These snack ideas and quick meal recipes are designed to be nutritious, easy to prepare, and suitable for individuals managing COPD. They provide a balance of protein, healthy fats, and carbohydrates to support energy levels and overall health. Adjust portion sizes and ingredients based on individual dietary needs and preferences.

CHAPTER FOUR
How Dehydration Affects Copd Symptoms

Dehydration can significantly affect COPD (Chronic Obstructive Pulmonary Disease) symptoms and overall health due to its impact on respiratory function and general well-being. Here are several ways dehydration can exacerbate COPD symptoms:

1. Increased Mucus Thickness:

• **Effect**: Dehydration reduces the body's ability to produce thin, watery mucus that helps keep the airways moist and clear.

• **Consequence**: Thicker mucus is harder to expel from the airways, leading to congestion, coughing, and difficulty breathing.

2. Reduced Mucus Clearance:

• **Effect**: Inadequate hydration can impair the cilia (small hair-like structures) in the airways that help move mucus out of the lungs.

• **Consequence**: This impairs the lungs' ability to clear mucus and debris, increasing the risk of respiratory infections and exacerbations.

3. Increased Respiratory Effort:

• **Effect**: Dehydration can lead to fluid loss throughout the body, including in the respiratory tract.

• **Consequence**: This loss can make breathing more difficult as the body works harder to maintain oxygen levels and remove carbon dioxide.

4. Worsened Fatigue and Weakness:

• **Effect**: Dehydration reduces overall energy levels and muscle function.

- **Consequence**: COPD patients already experience fatigue due to compromised lung function. Dehydration can exacerbate this fatigue, making daily activities more challenging.

5. Increased Risk of Exacerbations:

- **Effect**: Dehydration weakens the immune system and compromises lung function.

- **Consequence**: This increases the susceptibility to respiratory infections and exacerbations of COPD symptoms, leading to hospitalizations and worsening of the condition.

6. Impact on Medication Effectiveness:

- **Effect**: Some medications used to manage COPD, such as bronchodilators and corticosteroids, require adequate hydration to be effective.

• **Consequence**: Dehydration can reduce the effectiveness of these medications, potentially leading to inadequate symptom control.

Prevention and Management:

To prevent dehydration and its negative effects on COPD, it's essential for individuals to:

• **Monitor Fluid Intake**: Aim to drink plenty of fluids throughout the day, primarily water. Adjust intake based on activity level, weather conditions, and individual needs.

• **Limit Dehydrating Substances**: Reduce consumption of caffeinated beverages and alcohol, as they can increase fluid loss.

• **Hydrate Before and After Physical Activity**: Drink fluids before and after physical exertion to maintain hydration levels.

• **Monitor Urine Color**: A pale yellow color indicates adequate hydration, while darker urine may suggest dehydration.

Individuals with COPD should discuss specific hydration needs and strategies with their healthcare team, especially if managing medications or experiencing frequent exacerbations.

By maintaining adequate hydration, individuals with COPD can help manage symptoms more effectively, reduce the risk of exacerbations, and improve overall quality of life.

Eating Challenges For COPD Patients

COPD (Chronic Obstructive Pulmonary Disease) can present several eating challenges due to its impact on breathing, energy levels, and overall health. These challenges can affect nutritional intake and mealtime comfort for individuals with COPD. Here are some common eating challenges for COPD patients:

1. Dyspnea (Shortness of Breath):

• **Challenge**: Breathing difficulties make eating physically taxing, especially during meals that require chewing and swallowing.

• **Impact**: COPD patients may experience fatigue and discomfort, which can reduce appetite and lead to inadequate calorie intake.

2. Fatigue and Weakness:

• **Challenge**: COPD-related fatigue can make meal preparation and eating a daunting task.

• **Impact**: This may result in skipped meals or reliance on convenience foods that may not be nutritious, affecting overall health.

3. Reduced Appetite:

• **Challenge**: Medications, respiratory symptoms, and changes in taste and smell can diminish appetite.

• **Impact**: Inadequate calorie and nutrient intake can lead to weight loss, muscle wasting, and compromised immune function.

4. Swallowing Difficulties (Dysphagia):

• **Challenge**: COPD can weaken respiratory muscles, including those involved in swallowing.

• **Impact**: Difficulty swallowing (dysphagia) can lead to choking, aspiration, and fear of eating, affecting food choices and enjoyment.

5. Medication Side Effects:

• **Challenge**: Some medications used to manage COPD may cause gastrointestinal symptoms such as nausea or dry mouth.

• **Impact**: These side effects can further reduce appetite and affect taste perception, making it challenging to maintain adequate nutrition.

6. Dehydration:

• **Challenge**: COPD patients may avoid drinking fluids to reduce the need to urinate frequently or due to difficulty swallowing liquids.

Impact: Dehydration can worsen respiratory symptoms, increase mucus thickness, and compromise overall health.

7. Anxiety and Stress:

• **Challenge**: Anxiety related to breathing difficulties and COPD management can affect appetite and mealtime comfort.

• **Impact**: Stress can contribute to irregular eating patterns, poor food choices, and difficulty maintaining a balanced diet.

Strategies to Address Eating Challenges:

• **Small, Frequent Meals**: Opt for smaller, more frequent meals throughout the day to reduce the physical demand of eating and maintain energy levels.

• **Nutrient-Dense Foods**: Prioritize foods rich in protein, healthy fats, vitamins, and minerals to maximize nutritional intake during meals and snacks.

• **Easy-to-Prepare Meals**: Choose simple recipes that require minimal preparation and cooking time to conserve energy and reduce mealtime stress.

• **Hydration**: Drink fluids regularly throughout the day, and consider using a straw or sipping from a water bottle to make drinking easier.

• **Assistive Devices**: Use adaptive utensils, such as utensils with larger handles or a rocker knife, to make eating more manageable for those with limited strength or dexterity.

• **Meal Planning and Support**: Work with a dietitian or healthcare provider to create a personalized meal plan that addresses individual nutritional needs and challenges.

• **Medication Management**: Discuss medication schedules and potential side effects with healthcare providers to minimize their impact on appetite and eating habits.

• **Breathing Techniques**: Practice breathing exercises recommended by healthcare providers to improve lung function and reduce dyspnea during meals.

Addressing eating challenges in COPD requires a holistic approach that considers physical limitations, nutritional needs, and individual preferences. By implementing strategies to support eating comfort and nutritional intake, individuals with COPD can better manage symptoms and improve their overall quality of life.

CHAPTER FIVE
Lifestyle Tips For Better COPD Management

Managing COPD (Chronic Obstructive Pulmonary Disease) involves a comprehensive approach that goes beyond medical treatments. Here are lifestyle tips that can help individuals with COPD manage their condition effectively:

1. **Quit Smoking and Avoid Secondhand Smoke:**

• **Importance**: Smoking cessation is crucial in slowing disease progression and reducing symptoms. Avoiding secondhand smoke is also important.

• **Action**: Seek support from healthcare providers, join smoking cessation programs, and remove triggers that may lead to smoking relapse.

2. Stay Active with Regular Exercise:

• **Importance**: Physical activity improves lung function, strengthens respiratory muscles, and enhances overall endurance.

• **Action**: Engage in activities like walking, swimming, or stationary biking. Start slowly and gradually increase intensity under guidance from healthcare providers.

3. Maintain a Healthy Diet:

• **Importance**: Proper nutrition supports immune function, muscle strength, and overall well-being, which are crucial for COPD management.

• **Action**: Eat a balanced diet rich in fruits, vegetables, lean proteins, whole grains, and healthy fats. Avoid processed foods and excessive salt.

4. Hydrate Adequately:

- **Importance**: Good hydration helps keep mucus thin and easier to clear from the airways, reducing respiratory symptoms.

- **Action**: Drink plenty of water throughout the day. Limit caffeine and alcohol intake, as they can contribute to dehydration.

5. Practice Good Respiratory Hygiene:

- **Importance**: Preventing respiratory infections is key to managing COPD and avoiding exacerbations.

- **Action**: Wash hands frequently, avoid crowded places during flu season, and get vaccinated annually against influenza and pneumococcal infections.

6. Manage Stress Effectively:

- **Importance**: Stress can exacerbate COPD symptoms. Learning to manage stress can improve overall well-being.

• **Action**: Practice relaxation techniques such as deep breathing, meditation, yoga, or tai chi. Seek support from counselors or support groups if needed.

7. Monitor Symptoms and Medications:

• **Importance**: Regular monitoring helps track disease progression and ensures medications are effective.

• **Action**: Keep a symptom diary, attend regular follow-up appointments with healthcare providers, and adhere to prescribed medications and therapies.

8. Optimize Indoor Air Quality:

• **Importance**: Poor indoor air quality can worsen COPD symptoms. Ensuring a clean and allergen-free environment is essential.

• **Action**: Keep indoor spaces well-ventilated, use air purifiers if necessary, and avoid exposure to smoke, strong odors, and pollutants.

9. **Get Sufficient Sleep:**

• **Importance**: Quality sleep supports overall health and helps manage fatigue associated with COPD.

• **Action**: Maintain a regular sleep schedule, create a comfortable sleep environment, and practice good sleep hygiene habits.

10. **Educate Yourself and Seek Support:**

• **Importance**: Understanding COPD and its management empowers individuals to make informed decisions and advocate for their health.

• **Action**: Stay informed through reputable sources, participate in COPD education programs or support groups, and communicate openly with healthcare providers.

By incorporating these lifestyle tips into daily routines, individuals with COPD can enhance their quality of life, manage symptoms more effectively, and reduce the risk of exacerbations. Consistency and collaboration with healthcare providers are key to successful COPD management.

Breakfast Recipes Options

Here are some nutritious and easy-to-prepare breakfast recipes suitable for individuals managing COPD (Chronic Obstructive Pulmonary Disease). These recipes focus on providing balanced nutrition, supporting energy levels, and being easy to digest:

1. Oatmeal with Berries and Almonds:

Ingredients:

- 1/2 cup rolled oats
- 1 cup milk (dairy or plant-based)

- Handful of mixed berries (strawberries, blueberries, raspberries)
- 1 tablespoon chopped almonds or walnuts
- Optional: honey or maple syrup for sweetness

Instructions:

- In a small saucepan, bring milk to a boil.
- Stir in rolled oats and reduce heat to medium-low. Cook for 5-7 minutes, stirring occasionally, until oats are tender and creamy.
- Transfer oatmeal to a bowl. Top with mixed berries, chopped nuts, and a drizzle of honey or maple syrup if desired.

2. Yogurt Parfait:

Ingredients:

- 1/2 cup Greek yogurt (plain or flavored)
- 1/4 cup granola
- Handful of sliced strawberries or other fresh fruits
- Optional: a sprinkle of chia seeds or ground flaxseeds

Instructions:

- In a glass or bowl, layer Greek yogurt, granola, and sliced strawberries (or other fruits).
- Repeat layers until ingredients are used up.
- Top with a sprinkle of chia seeds or ground flaxseeds for added nutrition.

3. *Vegetable Omelette:*

Ingredients:

- 2 eggs
- Handful of spinach leaves

- 1/4 cup diced tomatoes

- 1/4 cup diced bell peppers (any color)

- 1/4 cup shredded cheese (such as cheddar or mozzarella)

- Salt and pepper to taste

- Optional: chopped herbs (like parsley or basil)

Instructions:

- In a bowl, whisk eggs with salt, pepper, and optional herbs.

- Heat a non-stick skillet over medium heat. Add spinach, tomatoes, and bell peppers, and cook until softened.

- Pour whisked eggs over the vegetables in the skillet. Cook until the edges start to set, then sprinkle shredded cheese evenly over the omelette.

- Fold the omelette in half and cook for another 1-2 minutes until cheese melts and eggs are fully cooked.

4. *Whole Grain Toast with Avocado and Poached Egg:*

Ingredients:

- 1 slice of whole grain bread, toasted
- 1/2 ripe avocado, mashed
- 1 poached egg
- Salt and pepper to taste
- Optional: a sprinkle of red pepper flakes or paprika

Instructions:

- Toast whole grain bread until golden brown.
- Spread mashed avocado evenly on the toast. Season with salt, pepper, and optional red pepper flakes or paprika.
- Top with a poached egg. Pierce the yolk to allow it to run over the avocado toast.

5. *Fruit Smoothie:*

Ingredients:

- 1/2 cup plain Greek yogurt
- 1/2 cup unsweetened almond milk (or any milk of choice)
- 1/2 banana, frozen
- Handful of spinach leaves
- 1/2 cup mixed berries (strawberries, blueberries, raspberries)
- Optional: 1 tablespoon honey or maple syrup for sweetness

Instructions:

• In a blender, combine Greek yogurt, almond milk, frozen banana, spinach, mixed berries, and optional honey or maple syrup.

• Blend until smooth and creamy. Add more almond milk if needed to achieve desired consistency.

These breakfast recipes are designed to be nutritious, easy to prepare, and tailored to support individuals managing COPD. They provide a balance of protein, healthy fats, fiber, vitamins, and minerals to help maintain energy levels and overall well-being. Adjust ingredients based on personal preferences and dietary needs.

Lunch And Dinner Recipes

Here are some nutritious and COPD-friendly lunch and dinner recipes that focus on providing balanced nutrition and supporting respiratory health:

Lunch Recipes:

1. Grilled Chicken Salad:

Ingredients:

- 4 oz grilled chicken breast, sliced
- Mixed salad greens (lettuce, spinach, arugula)
- 1/2 cucumber, sliced
- 1/2 cup cherry tomatoes, halved

- 1/4 cup sliced red onion

- 1/4 avocado, sliced

- Olive oil and balsamic vinegar for dressing

- Optional: sprinkle of feta cheese or nuts/seeds for added texture

Instructions:

• Arrange mixed salad greens on a plate.

• Top with grilled chicken breast, cucumber slices, cherry tomatoes, red onion, and avocado slices.

• Drizzle with olive oil and balsamic vinegar. Optionally, sprinkle with feta cheese or nuts/seeds.

2. Quinoa and Vegetable Stir-Fry:

Ingredients:

- 1/2 cup quinoa, rinsed

- 1 cup water or low-sodium vegetable broth
- 1 tablespoon olive oil
- 1/2 onion, thinly sliced
- 1 bell pepper (any color), thinly sliced
- 1 cup broccoli florets
- 1 carrot, sliced into matchsticks
- 2 tablespoons low-sodium soy sauce or tamari
- Optional: diced tofu or cooked chicken for added protein

Instructions:

- In a saucepan, combine quinoa and water or broth. Bring to a boil, then reduce heat to low. Cover and simmer for 15-20 minutes until quinoa is tender and water is absorbed.
- Heat olive oil in a large skillet or wok over medium-high heat. Add onion and cook until softened.

- Add bell pepper, broccoli, and carrot to the skillet. Stir-fry for 5-7 minutes until vegetables are tender-crisp.

- Stir in cooked quinoa and soy sauce or tamari. Add diced tofu or cooked chicken if using. Cook for another 2-3 minutes until heated through.

Dinner Recipes:

1. Baked Salmon with Sweet Potato Mash and Steamed Green Beans:

Ingredients:

- 4 oz salmon fillet
- 1 medium sweet potato, peeled and cubed
- 1 tablespoon olive oil
- Salt and pepper to taste
- 1 cup green beans, trimmed
- Lemon wedges for serving

Instructions:

• Preheat oven to 400°F (200°C).

• Place salmon fillet on a baking sheet lined with parchment paper. Drizzle with olive oil and season with salt and pepper. Bake for 15-20 minutes until salmon is cooked through and flakes easily with a fork.

• While salmon is baking, boil sweet potato cubes in a pot of water until tender, about 10-15 minutes. Drain and mash with a fork, adding a drizzle of olive oil and seasoning with salt and pepper.

• Steam green beans until tender-crisp, about 5 minutes.

• Serve baked salmon with sweet potato mash and steamed green beans. Squeeze lemon juice over salmon before serving.

2. *Turkey and Vegetable Stir-Fry:*

Ingredients:

- 4 oz turkey breast, sliced into strips

- 1 tablespoon olive oil

- 1/2 onion, thinly sliced

- 1 cup mixed vegetables (bell peppers, broccoli, snap peas)

- 2 tablespoons low-sodium soy sauce or tamari

- Cooked brown rice or quinoa for serving

Instructions:

• Heat olive oil in a large skillet or wok over medium-high heat. Add sliced turkey breast and cook until browned and cooked through, about 5-7 minutes. Remove from skillet and set aside.

• In the same skillet, add onion and cook until softened.

• Add mixed vegetables to the skillet and stir-fry for 5-7 minutes until tender-crisp.

• Return cooked turkey to the skillet. Stir in low-sodium soy sauce or tamari. Cook for another 2-3 minutes until heated through.

• Serve turkey and vegetable stir-fry over cooked brown rice or quinoa.

These lunch and dinner recipes are designed to be nutritious, easy to prepare, and tailored to support individuals managing COPD. They provide a balance of protein, healthy fats, fiber, vitamins, and minerals to help maintain energy levels and overall well-being. Adjust ingredients based on personal preferences and dietary needs.

Healthy Desserts And Snacks Recipes

Here are some healthy dessert and snack recipes that are suitable for individuals managing COPD (Chronic Obstructive Pulmonary Disease). These recipes focus on providing nutrient-dense options while being easy to prepare and enjoyable:

Healthy Dessert Recipes:

1. Mixed Berry Yogurt Popsicles:

Ingredients:

- 1 cup mixed berries (such as strawberries, blueberries, raspberries)
- 1 cup plain Greek yogurt
- 1-2 tablespoons honey or maple syrup (optional, depending on sweetness preference)
- Popsicle molds or small paper cups with popsicle sticks

Instructions:

• Blend mixed berries, Greek yogurt, and honey or maple syrup in a blender until smooth.

• Pour mixture into popsicle molds or small paper cups.

• Insert popsicle sticks into each mold.

Freeze for at least 4 hours or until fully set.

• Remove from molds and enjoy these refreshing yogurt popsicles.

2. **Baked Apples with Cinnamon and Walnuts:**

Ingredients:

- 2 apples (such as Granny Smith or Honeycrisp), cored
- 1 tablespoon chopped walnuts
- 1/2 teaspoon ground cinnamon
- 1 teaspoon honey or maple syrup
- Optional: a sprinkle of nutmeg or cloves

Instructions:

• Preheat oven to 375°F (190°C).

• Place cored apples on a baking sheet lined with parchment paper.

• In a small bowl, mix chopped walnuts, ground cinnamon, honey or maple syrup, and optional nutmeg or cloves.

• Spoon the walnut mixture into the center of each apple.

• Bake for 20-25 minutes until apples are tender and topping is golden brown.

• Serve warm as a healthy and comforting dessert.

Healthy Snack Recipes:

1. Chia Seed Pudding:

Ingredients:

- 1/4 cup chia seeds
- 1 cup unsweetened almond milk (or any milk of choice)
- 1 tablespoon honey or maple syrup
- Optional toppings: fresh berries, sliced bananas, chopped nuts

Instructions:

• In a bowl or jar, combine chia seeds, almond milk, and honey or maple syrup. Stir well.

• Cover and refrigerate for at least 2 hours or overnight until the mixture thickens and resembles pudding.

• Stir well before serving and top with fresh berries, sliced bananas, or chopped nuts for added flavor and texture.

<u>*2. Roasted Chickpeas:*</u>

Ingredients:

- 1 can (15 oz) chickpeas, drained and rinsed
- 1 tablespoon olive oil
- 1/2 teaspoon ground cumin
- 1/2 teaspoon smoked paprika
- Salt and pepper to taste

Instructions:

- Preheat oven to 400°F (200°C).
- Pat chickpeas dry with a paper towel to remove excess moisture.
- In a bowl, toss chickpeas with olive oil, ground cumin, smoked paprika, salt, and pepper until evenly coated.
- Spread chickpeas in a single layer on a baking sheet lined with parchment paper.

- Roast for 20-25 minutes, stirring halfway through, until chickpeas are crispy and golden brown.
- Allow to cool slightly before serving as a crunchy and protein-rich snack.

Tips for COPD-Friendly Desserts and Snacks:

• **Portion Control**: Enjoy desserts and snacks in moderate portions to avoid overeating.

• **Nutrient-Dense Choices**: Opt for snacks that provide fiber, protein, and healthy fats to promote satiety and sustained energy levels.

• **Hydration**: Pair snacks with water or herbal tea to stay hydrated, which is important for managing COPD symptoms.

• **Ingredient Modifications**: Adjust recipes to suit dietary preferences or restrictions, such as using dairy-free alternatives or reducing added sugars.

These dessert and snack recipes offer flavorful options that can be enjoyed while supporting a balanced diet for individuals managing COPD. They provide a mix of textures and flavors to satisfy cravings without compromising nutritional goals.

CHAPTER SIX
Eating Out And Traveling With COPD

Managing COPD (Chronic Obstructive Pulmonary Disease) while eating out or traveling requires planning and awareness to ensure comfort and proper nutrition. Here are some tips to navigate dining out and traveling with COPD:

Eating Out:

Choose Restaurants Wisely:

• Opt for restaurants that offer a variety of options, including lighter meals with grilled or steamed dishes.

• Look for menus that feature lean proteins (like grilled chicken or fish), whole grains, and plenty of vegetables.

Request Modifications:

• Don't hesitate to ask for modifications to suit your dietary needs, such as requesting sauces or dressings on the side, or substituting fries for a side salad or steamed vegetables.

Be Mindful of Portions:

• Restaurant portions are often larger than what you might eat at home. Consider sharing a dish with a dining partner or ask for a half portion to avoid overeating.

Avoid Trigger Foods:

• If certain foods or ingredients trigger COPD symptoms, such as dairy or spicy foods, choose alternatives that are gentler on your digestive and respiratory systems.

Stay Hydrated:

• Drink water or non-caffeinated beverages throughout the meal to stay hydrated. Avoid excessive alcohol consumption, which can dehydrate the body.

Take Your Time:

• Eating slowly and chewing thoroughly can aid digestion and reduce the risk of discomfort, especially if breathing is affected.

Traveling:

Plan Ahead:

• Research restaurants and grocery stores at your destination that offer healthy meal options or ingredients you can use to prepare meals in your accommodation.

Pack Snacks:

• Bring along portable, COPD-friendly snacks such as nuts, seeds, dried fruits, or whole grain crackers to have on hand during travel.

Medication and Supplies:

• Pack all necessary medications, inhalers, and medical supplies in your carry-on bag. Ensure you have enough for the duration of your trip, plus extra in case of delays.

Stay Active During Travel:

• If possible, take short walks or do stretching exercises during travel to keep circulation and lung function optimal.

Consider Air Quality:

• Pay attention to air quality alerts at your destination, especially if traveling to areas with high pollution levels or allergens that could exacerbate COPD symptoms.

Manage Stress:

• Traveling can be stressful, which may impact COPD symptoms. Practice relaxation techniques, such as deep breathing or meditation, to manage stress levels.

Stay Hydrated:

Air travel and changes in climate can lead to dehydration. Drink water regularly and avoid excessive caffeine or alcohol intake.

General Tips:

• **Communicate with Travel Companions:** Inform them about your condition and any specific needs or concerns you have regarding meals or activities.

• **Medical Alert Information:** Wear a medical alert bracelet or carry a card that outlines your COPD diagnosis, medications, and emergency contacts.

• **Travel Insurance:** Consider purchasing travel insurance that covers medical emergencies, including exacerbations of COPD or the need for medical evacuation.

By planning ahead, making mindful choices, and prioritizing your health needs, you can enjoy dining out and traveling while managing COPD effectively. It's important to listen to your body, pace yourself, and seek medical advice if you experience any worsening of symptoms during your travels.

Summary

A combination of medical treatment, behavioral changes, and attentive decision-making in everyday situations, as while dining out or traveling, is necessary for chronic obstructive pulmonary disease (COPD) management. You can enhance your quality of life and manage chronic obstructive pulmonary disease (COPD) by making the following changes to your daily routine:

• To keep your health under control, it is important to take your medicine as directed, see your doctor regularly, and be honest with them about any changes in your symptoms or worries.

• A Well-Rounded Way of Living: Eat plenty of fresh produce, lean meats, and whole grains to keep your diet well-rounded. Hydrate yourself, move around as much as you can safely, get enough sleep, and learn to control your stress.

• Being Conscious of the Environment: Pay attention to the air quality both inside and outside your home; stay away from anything that can aggravate respiratory problems, like smoke, pollutants, and allergies.

• Traveling with COPD: Do your homework on what restaurants are accommodating to people with the disease, make sure you have all of your meds and supplies on hand, and let your waiters or companions know what you need before you go.

• Reach out to loved ones, friends, and medical experts for emotional and practical help. You can find more encouragement and resources by joining a support group or an educational program.

Manage chronic obstructive pulmonary disease (COPD), reduce the frequency and severity of exacerbations, and live your life to the fullest by making these changes a regular part of your routine. Always keep in mind that your experience with chronic obstructive pulmonary disease (COPD) is unique, and adjust these tactics accordingly.

Optimize your journey with chronic obstructive pulmonary disease (COPD) by being proactive in your self-care and seeking help from healthcare professionals when needed.

THE END

www.ingramcontent.com/pod-product-compliance
Lightning Source LLC
Chambersburg PA
CBHW061250250726
48653CB00002B/591